CONTENT

CW00401364

Chapter 1: Understanding t Weight Gain

Chapter 2: The Truth About Processed Foods

Chapter 3: Re-thinking the Calorie Myth

Chapter 4: Transforming Your Mental Health

VERIFIED REVIEWS FROM CLIENTS

Adrian Burman

"Stefano keeps you motivated and accountable throughout and his knowledge is unmatched. The material you get alone is worth so much and leaves no stone unturned. Stefano knows what you need to do to maintain and keep the weight off long term, which is where all the other systems fail. This is the only program you need to succeed and succeed you will if you commit to what Stefano sets out for you."

Steve Jackson

"Had the pleasure of taking part in UDT a few years ago, taught me some very good lessons and insights and more importantly I lost 50lbs and felt great. Stef and the guys were always available to chat and help!"

James Fitzpatrick-Ellis

"The program is amazing and really does work! It works, not only because of the program, but also because of the community of committed Dads, but because Coach is continually researching and learning about the core subjects that are involved.

Neil Mateer

"Can't recommend the UDT program highly enough. Great education, support and accountability resulting in good success. I was able to lose 26lbs in 12weeks."

Simon Jenner

"I did UDT 5 years ago and lost 4 stone in 90 days. It was life changing. great from start to finish Stefano is an excellent coach and very motivational, he wants you to succeed and will hold you accountable."

Roy Medlam

"Ultimate dad is by far the best health and fitness program I've ever come across Stefano goes above and beyond to help his clients reach their goals highly recommended."

Alan Calvert

"Stefano is not only knowledgeable and patient but also understands what the 'real world' is and the challenges that it brings to us in our everyday life's.

This is not just a weight loss programme (and it does achieve that) this is a lifestyle change that will leave you feeling better in all aspects of your life."

Jon Morecroft

"No quick fixes and no gimmicks - this is a lifestyle change that works. I completed the 12-week programme and followed it up with a further year of weight loss work as I moved through Stefano's brilliant plans. This resulted in me losing over 40kg!"

Andy McAllan

"100% recommend UDT and Stefano. He supports you 100%along the way and doesn't try to sell you any snake oil methods. He knows his stuff and isn't afraid to tell you how it is."

Martin Bertram

"This program really is a great way to lose weight that you've been having trouble doing. I started wanting to lose 10kg's that by going to the gym 3 days a week couldn't budge it. I lost my target (10kg's) in the 12-week program."

Andy King

This guy knows! Of all the things I've tried, there's one that really works if you follow the plan. Stefano provides a plan that covers nutrition, training and mindset and gets results!

Steve Bullock

"Fantastic programme to join if you're looking to lose weight & completely transform yourself, I joined & completed the 12 weeks programme."

Alan Barry

"Started UDT as a sceptic weighing nearly 20 stone. currently sitting just below 16 stone and it is entirely due to Stefano and the rest of the dads in here. I'm fitter, healthier, and eating better than I have ever done."

FOREWORD BY THE AUTHOR

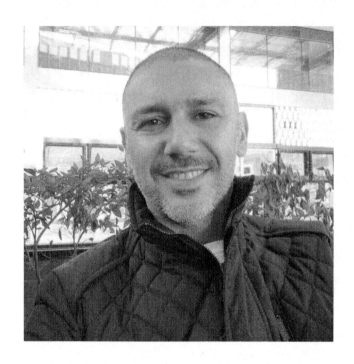

According to Cancer Research UK (CRUK), more than 42 million UK adults will be obese by 2040 (1), and it's a growing concern. The British Heart Foundation also reported that 7.6 million people are living with heart and circulatory diseases, with someone being admitted to the hospital every 5 minutes due to a stroke (2).

Mental health is also a big issue in the UK, with 1 in 4 people experiencing mental health problems according to mind.org (3), and even children are being affected, with a 39% increase according to NHS 2023 data (4), learning how to take better care of your body and mind should now be considered essential reading.

Relying on the government and the NHS to save us is a recipe for disaster, as doctor and hospital appointments are becoming harder to come by. The solution is to educate ourselves and become self-sufficient to protect our health and our families, becoming a rolemodel and leader for them.

The weight loss industry is worth billions that promise quick and easy solutions to our weight struggles that fail to provide a competent solution. From fad diets to weight loss supplements, the industry is constantly trying to sell us new products with promises of fast weight loss, but the reality is that these approaches often fail to deliver the results we want.

Exercise is a traditional approach to weight loss, but it's not practical for busy dads who don't have the time and energy to commit to long-term exercise. It can also be monotonous, leading to feelings of burnout and lack of motivation.

That's why I created a book specifically for busy dads who want to take back control of their health, weight, body, and life. If you're tired of feeling tired, overweight, and stressed out, tired of trying every diet and exercise program out there without seeing results, and lacking motivation, I understand how you feel. I've been there myself.

I remember feeling overweight, tired, and lacking energy for my family. I felt like a failure and didn't like the person I saw in the mirror. I was putting everyone else first but neglecting my own health, and every failed attempt to change only made me feel worse. Processed foods, alcohol, takeaways, and a lack of movement became the norm for me under the excuse of not having enough time.

I realized that my pride and ego were holding me back from admitting that I had a problem. The truth is, you can't pour from an empty cup, and I was telling myself lies that it was okay to not have energy for my kids, that I was shortening my life, or that my wife wouldn't find me attractive anymore. I had to change my mindset and focus on the opportunity to become better, rather than the struggle.

So, I took full ownership and became mentally fit and strong. I rediscovered my love for my family and my own self-love, and now I want to help you do the same. I want to show you how to turn your story around, the right way.

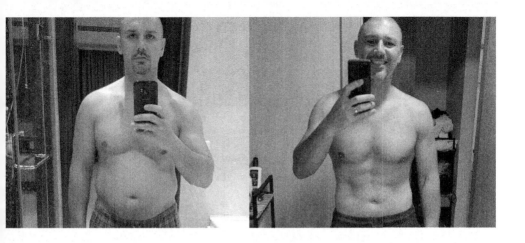

I wrote a book specifically for people like you who are tired of trying the same weight loss methods repeatedly without any lasting success.

I'm here to share the truth about the weight loss industry and why counting calories and long-term exercise just aren't cutting it. We'll get to the bottom of why you're struggling with weight gain, like stress, lack of sleep, hormone imbalances, and how the food industry is making it even harder for you.

I'll help you break through the calorie myth and show you the truth about processed foods. Plus, we'll work on transforming your mental health and ditching those excuses once and for all.

And when you hit those plateaus, I've got you covered. I'll show you how to stay motivated and make this weight loss journey a lifestyle change that will stick with you for good.

Some of the information in the book may challenge what you've learned before, but don't worry, I'll set the record straight. I've been coaching for 20 years and have helped over 1,000 dads just like you transform their lives. This book is based on the core principles of my coaching program and I promise it's packed with the latest and most relevant information to help you change your life this year and beyond! So, don't skip a chapter. I can't wait for you to start reading and transforming your life!

STEFANO 'THE DAD COACH' CHIRIACO

Previously Great Britain's Official PT Of the Year (IFS Awards) as seen in Men's Health, Men's Fitness & more.

Founder of 'Ultimate Dad Transformation', the 'Ultimate Dad Podcast' and 'The 90 Day Fit Dad Accelerator Programme'.

1000+ Dads Transformed losing 10-20 KG in less than 90 days with 20+ successful years in the coaching industry.

Contact: stefano@ultimatedadtransformation.com
Website: www.ultimatedadtransformation.com

Chapter 1: Understanding the Root Cause of Weight Gain

So, I know you're probably feeling overwhelmed about your weight. The good news is, you're not alone. Many men struggle with weight gain and it's a complex issue that can be caused by a variety of factors.

For starters, if you're taking in more calories than you're burning, that excess is getting stored as fat and causing weight gain. This can happen from eating a lot of processed and sugary foods, as well as a lack of physical activity and exercise.

And, unfortunately, genetics can also play a role in your weight. Certain genes can increase your risk of becoming overweight or obese, affecting your appetite, metabolism, and fat storage.

Even hormones can play a part, with changes in hormones as we age leading to weight gain for many men.

Now, here's the important part - weight gain isn't always a result of poor choices or lifestyle habits. It's a complex issue that requires a multi-faceted approach to address.

So don't worry, in this chapter, we'll dive deeper into the causes of weight gain specifically for men and explore ways to manage it effectively. Sound good?

Biological Factors

Have you ever wondered why it feels like no matter what you do, you just can't seem to lose weight? Well, the truth is, hormones play a big role in regulating your weight and metabolism. When your hormones are imbalanced, it can lead to weight gain.

For example, insulin is a hormone that helps control your blood sugar levels. But when insulin levels get too high, your body stores fat instead of burning it (5), leading to weight gain. If you have insulin resistance, which means your body is less sensitive to insulin, you may have higher insulin levels and be at a higher risk of weight gain.

To help regulate insulin levels, it's important to eat a healthy diet low in processed foods, added sugars, and refined carbs, and high in fiber, lean protein, and healthy fats. And don't forget to exercise regularly to improve insulin sensitivity.

Another hormone to watch out for is cortisol, the stress hormone. When cortisol levels are high, it can cause weight gain and disrupt your sleep. To lower cortisol levels, try doing stress-reducing activities like yoga or meditation, and make sure to get enough sleep each night.

Your thyroid gland also affects your weight. It produces hormones that regulate your metabolism, but if it doesn't produce enough, it can slow down and cause weight gain. Eating a diet rich in iodine, selenium, and zinc, and exercising regularly can help improve thyroid function.

It's worth noting that hormones imbalances can be caused by many things, like genetics, stress, poor diet, lack of sleep, and certain medications. Finding and fixing the root cause is key to managing weight gain.

And if you want to try a more natural approach, there are supplements like magnesium, omega-3 fatty acids, chromium, and probiotics that can help improve hormone imbalances. But before making any changes, it's best to talk to a healthcare professional, especially if you have any existing medical conditions or are unsure about the safety of a particular supplement.

The impact of genetics

I want to share some information with you about the impact of genetics on weight loss.

First, it's well-known that genetics (6) play a major role in our body weight and the likelihood of gaining or losing weight. One of the ways this happens is through the regulation of our metabolism and appetite. Some genetic variations are associated with increased hunger and a slower metabolism, making it harder for people to control their calorie intake and burn off excess energy.

Aside from the direct effects on weight loss, genetics can also impact weight loss indirectly by affecting lifestyle factors like physical activity and diet. For instance, some genetic variations are linked to reduced motivation for physical activity, which can lead to weight gain. Similarly, certain genetic variations can impact food preferences, making it harder for those individuals to stick to a healthy diet.

It's important to remember that genetics aren't the only things influencing weight loss. Other things like lifestyle, environment, and culture also play a major role.

So, what does this mean for you and your weight loss journey? Understanding the impact of genetics on weight loss can help you tailor a weight loss strategy that's right for you. For example, if you have genetic variations that make it harder to control your calorie intake and metabolism, you may need to be extra mindful of your calorie intake and focus on high-intensity exercise to burn more calories.

It's also important to consider your body type when developing a weight loss plan. For example, if you have an endomorph body type, you have a larger body frame and tend to store fat easily, so focusing on high-intensity exercise and a low-carb diet might be the best approach for you. On the other hand, if you have an ectomorph body type with a smaller frame, you may struggle to gain weight, so focusing on strength training and a higher-carb diet to build muscle mass and increase metabolism might be more appropriate.

In conclusion, genetics play a significant role in weight loss, but it's important to consider other factors like lifestyle, environment, and culture as well. Understanding the impact of genetics on weight loss can help you create an effective and sustainable weight loss plan that's right for you.

The Role of Gut Health And Metabolism In Weight Gain

Recent studies have shown that gut health plays a crucial role in weight gain and metabolism.

Scientists took bacteria from identical human twins where one was obese and one was lean, transferred them into lean mice and found that the mice with the 'fat' gut bacteria gained weight (7). This shows you that you must pay attention to this part of your health to succeed.

The gut microbiome is like a whole ecosystem inside of our body and it has a significant impact on our weight and metabolism. It can control our appetite, help with nutrient absorption, and also regulate insulin sensitivity.

Did you know that people with a more diverse gut microbiome tend to have better appetite regulation, which helps them control their weight better? And, a healthy gut microbiome can also improve nutrient absorption, which in turn helps maintain a healthy metabolism.

Another way gut health affects weight gain and metabolism is through the production of short-chain fatty acids (SCFAs). SCFAs are produced when gut bacteria ferment fiber, and they play a crucial role in maintaining a healthy gut barrier and regulating energy metabolism. But, a lack of SCFAs can lead to increased inflammation and insulin resistance, which can contribute to weight gain and other health issues.

So, how can we maintain or improve gut health? Well, it all starts with our diet. A diet high in processed foods, sugar, and saturated fats can promote the growth of harmful bacteria and lead to inflammation, while a diet high in fiber, fruits, and vegetables can promote the growth of beneficial bacteria. That's why incorporating more fiber, fruits and veggies in our diet can have a positive impact on our gut health.

In addition to dietary changes, natural supplements like probiotics, prebiotics and fiber can also help improve gut health. Exercise, stress management, and adequate sleep are also essential for maintaining a healthy gut microbiome. Regular physical activity has been shown to improve gut barrier function and reduce inflammation, while chronic stress and sleep deprivation can disrupt the gut microbiome and contribute to weight gain.

So, as you can see, maintaining a healthy gut is important for weight loss and overall health. By incorporating dietary changes, natural supplements, exercise, stress management, and adequate sleep, we can improve our gut health and achieve our weight loss goals.

Psychological Factors

Let's talk about stress, as it's a major contributor to weight gain (8) and can have a significant impact on your overall health and well-being.

When stress becomes chronic, it can cause hormonal imbalances in your body. The primary hormone affected by stress is cortisol, the "stress hormone". When cortisol levels are elevated, it can cause an increase in appetite and cravings for high-calorie, high-fat foods, leading to weight gain.

Furthermore, cortisol can also promote fat storage, especially in the abdominal area, something I'm sure you'd like to avoid. Another way stress can contribute to weight gain is by disrupting your metabolism, leading to a slower metabolism and reduced fat burning. Chronic stress has also been linked to insulin resistance, which can contribute to weight gain and other related health issues.

Stress can also cause disruptions in your sleep patterns, leading to sleep deprivation. When you don't get enough sleep, your body releases the hormone ghrelin, which stimulates appetite, and less of the hormone leptin, which controls appetite and energy. This can lead to further weight gain.

That's why it's so important to manage your stress levels, and there are many ways to do this. Exercise, such as running or lifting weights, can help release endorphins, which are natural mood elevators, and burn off stress-related cortisol. Yoga and meditation can also be effective in reducing stress and promoting relaxation and mindfulness.

Taking deep breaths and practicing deep breathing exercises can also help manage stress by slowing down your body's stress response and promoting relaxation.

And don't forget about the power of leisure activities such as reading, spending time with friends and family, or listening to music. They can also help to manage stress and bring you a sense of joy and happiness.

It's also crucial to pay attention to your diet, as a diet high in processed foods and sugar can contribute to inflammation and weight gain. Make sure to incorporate plenty of fruits and vegetables into your diet, and avoid processed foods and high amounts of sugar.

In conclusion, managing stress is an essential part of maintaining a healthy weight and overall well-being. Try incorporating some of these stress-management techniques into your daily routine and see the positive impact it has on your health and weight!

The Connection Between Emotional Eating and Weight

I understand that you might be struggling with emotional eating. It's a common issue where we tend to eat not because we're hungry, but because of our emotional state - be it stress, boredom, sadness, or even happiness.

According to a study done by the National Library of Medicine, emotional eaters consume more food under stress and gain relief from it (10).

This type of eating can be a response to a wide range of feelings, such as stress, boredom, sadness, and even happiness. Unfortunately, emotional eating can lead to some serious health consequences, including weight gain.

One of the main reasons why emotional eating contributes to weight gain is because of the poor food choices we make when we're feeling an emotional trigger. Often, the foods we crave when we're feeling an emotion are high in calories, high in fat, and very tempting. These types of foods can activate the pleasure centres in our brain, making it difficult to stop eating once we've started.

Another way emotional eating can impact our weight is by interfering with our ability to recognize and respond to our body's natural hunger and fullness signals. When we're eating in response to our emotions, we're less likely to pay attention to the cues our body is sending us about how much food we need. This can cause us to eat more than our body needs, leading to weight gain over time.

Stress is another factor that can contribute to weight gain through emotional eating. When we're feeling stressed, our bodies release cortisol, which is a stress hormone. Cortisol can cause us to feel more hungry and crave higher calorie, high-fat foods, which can make it even more challenging to avoid emotional eating.

To help manage emotional eating and prevent weight gain, it's essential to get to the root of the problem. This can be done by keeping a food and mood diary, which can help you identify the emotions and situations that trigger your emotional eating. By understanding the underlying causes of your emotional eating, you can develop strategies to address it.

One strategy is to find healthy alternatives to your trigger foods. For example, instead of reaching for a pint of ice cream when you're feeling sad, you could opt for some unsweetened yogurt with fruit. Or, instead of snacking on chips when you're bored, you could grab some sliced carrots instead.

Another effective strategy is to practice mindful eating. This involves being present and attentive when you're eating, paying attention to the taste and texture of your food, and being aware of your body's hunger and fullness cues. Mindful eating can help you make healthier food choices and prevent overeating, reducing the risk of weight gain due to emotional eating.

The Role of Negative Self-talk And Beliefs in Weight

Let's cover something that is often overlooked, it's all about your self-talk and beliefs, and how they can greatly affect your weight loss journey.

According to the National Library of Medicine, significant associations were found between higher BMI and increased self-criticism (9).

First, let me talk about motivation and willpower. When we have negative thoughts about ourselves, it can be tough to stick to a healthy diet and exercise plan. It can leave you feeling unmotivated, hopeless, and defeated, making it easier to give in to unhealthy cravings and food choices.

Additionally, negative self-talk and beliefs can raise your stress levels, leading to higher cortisol levels. This in turn increases your appetite, triggers cravings for unhealthy foods, and promotes fat storage, especially around your abdominal area. Therefore it's crucial to be aware of our self-talk and challenge it.

As I always tell my clients, "The most powerful story in our lives is the one we tell ourselves every single day." So, by reframing negative thoughts, you can change the story you tell yourself and improve your motivation, willpower, and overall health.

For example, instead of saying "This is too hard," try saying "This is challenging, it makes me stronger." Instead of saying "I don't feel like exercising," try saying "I may not be in the mood, but I know I'll feel amazing after." And instead of saying "Why can't I lose weight?" try reframing it as "I have lost weight before and I can do it again if I keep going."

Moreover, negative self-talk and beliefs can also harm your self-esteem and body image, leading to neglect of self-care and ultimately weight gain. That's why it's important to practice self-compassion, being kind, understanding and forgiving towards yourself. Surrounding yourself with positive and supportive people and engaging in activities that bring you joy can also boost your mood, reduce stress, and contribute to your overall health and well-being.

Environmental Factors

With work, family, and other responsibilities, I know how easy it can be to spend hours sitting down each day. Unfortunately, that sedentary lifestyle is having a significant impact on your health, and I want to make sure you're aware of it.

First, sitting for long periods of time can lead to weight gain, as it burns fewer calories. In fact, every hour spent sitting reduces our energy expenditure, making it harder for you to burn calories and maintain a healthy weight. Prolonged sitting can also cause muscle atrophy, which can slow down your metabolism even further.

But it's not just your weight that's at risk. A sedentary lifestyle is also having a big impact on your heart health. Sitting for long periods of time has been linked to an increased risk of heart disease, high blood pressure, and diabetes. This is because sitting for long periods of time can cause your blood vessels to constrict, reducing blood flow to your heart and increasing the risk of blood clots. And the more time you spend in a chair, the greater the risk of death.

And let's not forget about your mental health. Sitting for long periods of time can lead to feelings of boredom, depression, and anxiety. And, a lack of physical activity has been linked to an increased risk of cognitive decline and dementia.

So, what can you do to manage the impact of a sedentary lifestyle on your health?

Well, first, make sure you incorporate regular physical activity into your daily routine. Aim for at least 30 minutes of moderate-intensity physical activity most days of the week, whether that be walking, cycling, swimming, or circuits/resistance exercise. Start slowly and gradually increase the intensity and duration of your physical activity over time.

Additionally, breaking up prolonged sitting by taking regular breaks throughout the day to stand up and move around can be extremely helpful. This can include taking a short walk, stretching, or doing some light exercises to increase blood flow and reduce the negative effects of prolonged sitting.

The food that is readily available to us also plays a huge role, namely processed foods which will be covered in chapter 2.

Diet Trends In 2023

You might have heard about the ketogenic diet, intermittent fasting, the vegan diet, and the all-meat diet. But the truth is, these diets are often marketed as quick fixes for weight loss and health, but, they can be difficult to maintain and may not be effective for everyone.

The ketogenic diet, or "keto" diet, is a high-fat, low-carbohydrate diet that puts your body into a state where it burns fat for energy instead of carbs. The idea behind it is that eliminating carbs will make your body switch from using glucose to using ketones produced by the liver when fat is broken down.

While it may help with initial water weight loss and some fat loss, it can also be hard to follow, as you need to eat 70% fat and strictly limit carbs. This high-fat intake may also lead to muscle loss due to a lack of protein (11), and lower energy levels, making it harder to exercise. The keto diet can also cause fatigue, irritability, constipation, and other symptoms, especially when trying to exercise. High-intensity exercise can't be sustained without carbs, limiting your ability to build muscle and maintain results in the long term.

Intermittent fasting is a pattern of eating that involves alternating periods of fasting and eating. The 16/8 method is the most popular one, where you fast for 16 hours and eat during an 8-hour window. While it may help with weight loss, many people end up overeating or binge eating during the eating window, which can counteract the benefits of fasting and even lead to weight gain. Intermittent fasting may also not be suitable for individuals with certain medical conditions and may not be sustainable for most people.

The vegan diet involves eating only plant-based foods and avoiding all animal products. Eating more vegetables is always a good thing, but the problem is that it requires a significant change in eating habits, limits eating out and can be expensive. Vegan diets may also lead to nutrient deficiencies if not planned properly, especially for proteins, iron, calcium, Vitamin D, and Vitamin B12. Plant-based proteins are less effective in the body compared to animal proteins, making it harder to hit protein targets and maintain muscle mass. A high intake of lectins in a vegan diet can also cause issues with digestion and malnutrition according to The National Library of Medicine (12).

The all-meat diet, or carnivore diet, consists only of animal products like meat, fish, dairy, and eggs. Some proponents argue that it promotes weight loss, improves energy levels and mental clarity, and improves certain health markers. However, it's not recommended by nutrition experts and health organizations, as it may lead to nutrient deficiencies and increase the risk of heart disease and certain cancers due to the high saturated fat and cholesterol content.

You might think you've lost weight using these diets, but the truth is, over 90% of people gain it back. The real question is, do these diets really work? When someone switches from processed foods to any of these diets, they're likely to lose weight, but this is only because they've eliminated the "bad food." Any change in nutrition habits from processed foods will result in improvement, but is it sustainable or healthy?

The evidence shows that diets don't work unless they're sustainable and long-term elimination of ANY food group is not the way to go when it comes to your health.

Short-term restriction or food elimination can work and even be beneficial, but unless there's a plan for sustainability, the results don't last, and that's where everyone struggles.

In conclusion, these diets may have some benefits, but they're often marketed as quick fixes for weight loss and overall health. It's important to remember that a healthy diet is balanced and includes a variety of nutrient-rich foods.

How Covid Changed Fitness

With the rise of online health and wellness options, it's becoming easier to get the information and support you need from the comfort of your own home. However, there's also a lot of conflicting information out there, so it can be difficult to know who to trust.

The good news is that there are now more options available, but the downside is that many of the online coaches out there may not be qualified professionals. They may have gained their qualifications in just a matter of weeks, which is concerning.

Personal trainers may only have basic knowledge of exercise and dietary advice, and they may not have the background or education to provide you with sound advice on how to live your life.

So, it's important to work with a qualified professional who takes a holistic approach to health and wellness. They should consider all factors, not just exercise and calorie counting. A good coach will also consider sustainability, mindset, personal growth, and accountability in helping you achieve and maintain a healthy lifestyle.

Your coach should take the time to understand your unique needs, goals, and challenges and work with you to create a plan that's sustainable and achievable. Also, be aware that some fitness professionals may use steroids, which can be misleading. It's always a good idea to do your research before working with anyone.

Remember, personal trainers are not qualified nutritionists or certified life coaches in most cases. So, if you're looking for guidance on nutrition, lifestyle, or overall well-being, it's best to work with someone who has specific education or training in those areas and is properly qualified.

In conclusion, it's important to ignore the noise and hype online. With the information you'll learn in this book, you'll be on the road to long-term success so you can achieve your health and fitness goals in a sustainable, rewarding, and enjoyable way.

Chapter 2: The Truth About Processed Foods

What Are Processed Foods?

You're probably feeling overwhelmed by all the information out there about what to eat and what not to eat. I'm here to simplify it for you and make sure you understand the effects of the Western diet.

The Western diet is filled with processed foods, saturated fats, sugar, and red meat, and has been linked to several serious health conditions like obesity, diabetes, and others. In countries where the Western diet has been adopted, rates of these conditions have increased dramatically. For example, Mexico has seen a huge jump in obesity, from 8% in 1988 to 32.4% in 2016 (13), making it the most obese country in the world. China is experiencing a similar trend, with obesity rates rising at an alarming rate (14).

A recent study in the Lancet [the oldest peer reviewed medical journal] found that high consumption of red meat, processed meat, sugary drinks, and trans fats was responsible for 11 million deaths worldwide in 2017 (15). This shows just how dangerous the Western diet can be for our health.

The story of how the Western diet became popular starts with the US government and the American Heart Association (AHA) back in the 1970s. They developed dietary guidelines that said reducing saturated fat was the key to preventing heart disease. This was based on a study called the Seven Countries Study, which only looked at a small group of men from seven countries and didn't consider other important dietary factors like added sugars, refined carbohydrates, and processed foods.

In recent years, many studies have challenged the findings of the Seven Countries Study and the idea that saturated fat is the main cause of heart disease. These new studies suggest that other dietary factors like added sugars, refined carbohydrates, and processed foods may play a bigger role in heart disease.

You see, many organizations, including the NHS, have been slow to update their guidelines and they still promote reducing saturated fat intake as the main way to prevent heart disease. But this has not been effective in helping people lose weight or improve their health.

Unfortunately, the NHS still promotes old methods which are not sustainable and can lead to weight regain with their latest program based around meal replacement shakes which is another form of starvation and a quick fix.

The issue with processed foods is that they've been altered from their natural state, usually with preservatives, artificial colours and flavours, or other ingredients. Examples of processed foods are frozen dinners, canned soups, and packaged snacks.

The rise of processed foods is due to several factors, like advances in food technology, changing consumer preferences, and the increasing demand for convenience. And, with the advances in food technology in the 1970s, mass producing processed foods on a large scale became possible and affordable for consumers.

Unfortunately, with the increased availability of processed foods, there was also a rise in weight gain among the population. Processed foods are often high in calories, sugar, and unhealthy fats, which can contribute to weight gain when consumed in excess. And they often lack fiber, vitamins, and minerals that are found in whole foods, making it harder to feel full and satisfied after eating.

Eating an orange has more fiber and nutrients than drinking orange juice and eating whole foods, like fruits, vegetables, whole grains, lean proteins, and healthy fats, will benefit your body more as they require more "processing" in the body, which burns more energy through digestion, helping with weight loss and a healthier metabolism.

Weight loss programs, like Slimming World and Weight Watchers, and supplement companies, often promote a calorie-restrictive approach to weight loss, but this has been criticized for promoting processed foods and a restrictive mindset towards food, leading to disordered eating patterns and an unhealthy relationship with food.

Rather than restrictive diets, it's better to focus on a balanced, nutrient-rich diet that includes a variety of fruits, vegetables, whole grains, lean proteins, and healthy fats, and to also have regular physical activity, good sleep, and stress management.

The evidence is clear, obesity and poor health have been driven by processed foods, restrictive diets that lack proper nourishment, and poor lifestyle habits due to the modern world.

The Industry's Misleading Claims

According to Grand View Research [2021], the global supplement industry was valued at 151 billion dollars and is only going to grow bigger! (16).

So before you start spending your hard-earned money on these products, let me give you the facts about what you need to know.

First, when it comes to weight loss, you might have heard that some supplements can help you burn fat or lose weight. And while it's true that some supplements like green tea extract or caffeine have been shown to have a small impact on weight loss, most of them don't have enough scientific evidence to support these claims. In fact, some of these products might even contain unproven ingredients or dosages that could be harmful to your health.

The same goes for supplements that claim to help you build muscle or improve your athletic performance. While some supplements like protein powder or creatine have been shown to have a small impact on muscle growth and athletic performance, most supplements don't have enough scientific evidence to support these claims. And once again, some of these products might contain unproven ingredients or dosages that could be harmful to your health.

When it comes to overall health and well-being, you might have heard that some supplements can improve your health. But, be careful, as many of these claims aren't backed by scientific evidence and can be misleading. Most of the vitamins and minerals that you need for good health can be obtained through a balanced diet, and taking too many supplements can actually be harmful to your health.

Now, you might be wondering, "Is the supplement industry regulated?" The answer is yes, but not in the way that you think. Supplement manufacturers can't make claims about how their products prevent, cure, or treat a condition, and very few supplements meet the criteria to obtain a medicinal claim license. Despite this, claims are still made and promised, and it will only ever be challenged if someone decides to report them.

Research shows that supplements are not actually making people healthier. In fact, a recent study showed that those people who already lead a healthy lifestyle (e.g. those who exercise and who are more conscious about what they eat) tend to be the ones taking nutritional supplements, making supplements appear to be health promoting by default. And a recent position statement from the British Medical Journal concluded that the current evidence does not support recommending vitamin or fish oil supplements to reduce the risk of non-communicable diseases among populations without clinical nutritional deficiency.

So, in conclusion, adults are spending so much money on supplements and probably not getting any real benefit from them. Before you start taking supplements, do your own research and use your own common sense. Make sure that you're getting your nutrients from a balanced diet, and if you still want to take supplements, be careful of the claims that the companies make and the ingredients that they contain.

The Impact of Marketing & Consumer Choices

According to a new survey (17), did you know that the UK consumes 4 times more processed foods than any other country in Europe? That's a lot of unhealthy food!

Have you ever stopped to think about how the food industry influences your purchasing decisions? Well, let me tell you, it's more than you think.

The food industry spends billions of dollars on advertising each year to make their products appealing to consumers like you and me. They use various tactics to make their products seem more desirable, such as celebrity endorsements and false health claims.

One tactic used by the food industry is targeting children and teens using colourful packaging, cartoon characters, and other techniques to make their products seem fun and exciting. But, what they don't tell you is that many of the foods marketed to kids are high in sugar, fat, and calories, which contributes to the growing problem of childhood obesity.

Another tactic the food industry uses is making false health claims about their products. For example, a company may claim that a food is "low-fat" or "organic" when it's not. This can lead you to believe that you're making a healthier choice, when, you're not.

Here is a breakdown of what food labels really mean:

Organic: You may think that organic means 'good for you' but it just means the food was made in another way and it doesn't mean it's healthier or less in calories.

Health Boosting 'Superfood': There is no actual definition or regulation around this but it's very effective at influencing your choices.

Low Fat: In the UK, it means the food has 3g of fat per 100g, but fat will be replaced with sugar. Whenever something is removed, something else will be added in. These high sugar swaps lead to overeating.

Low-Sugar: No added sugar doesn't mean it's low in sugar, check the labels!

Natural: This is very mis-leading, the food label may say it contains carrot concentrate

As you can see, the food industry also profits from promoting highly processed foods, which are often high in sugar, fat, and calories, and are cheap to produce. These processed foods are sold at a higher profit margin compared to healthier options, making them heavily advertised and promoted in supermarkets.

Not only that, but the food industry is capitalizing on the popularity of vegan options. They promote heavily processed vegan options, which can be high in calories, fat, and sodium, and may not offer the same nutritional benefits as whole plant-based foods.

The food industry is also known for promoting food products high in sugar and salt to increase cravings and make us want more – it's their 'marketing trick'. It's a vicious cycle that they benefit from, while we suffer the consequences.

Have you ever noticed how advertisements for food products often show fit models or people using exercise equipment? This is another tactic the industry uses to trick us into thinking that their product is beneficial, it's false advertising!

In conclusion, the food industry profits from promoting unhealthy food options, including vegan options, and uses misleading tactics to influence consumer behaviour. From false health claims to celebrity endorsements and misleading packaging, the food industry will do whatever it takes to make a profit, even if it means tricking us into thinking that we're making healthy choices.

The Impact of Processed Foods on Weight Gain

Have you ever considered the impact of processed foods on your weight gain despite even being low calorie?

The biggest trick that has been played on us all is that we have become obsessed with calories instead of food quality.

It's an important topic to discuss, as processed foods are everywhere and often make up a large part of our diets.

Let's start with added sugars. Have you ever checked the labels of the food you're buying? You may be surprised to see how much added sugar is in your food. In the UK, the average person consumes between 50-70g of added sugar per day, which is equivalent to 16 teaspoons! That's a lot of sugar! And it's not just in sweet treats like cakes and cookies, it's in things like salad dressings and sauces too.

Excessive consumption of added sugars can lead to weight gain, as well as a host of other health problems like diabetes, heart disease, and cancer. It's important to be aware of how much added sugar you're consuming and to make informed choices about the food you eat.

Now let's talk about sodium. Have you ever tasted processed food that was too salty? That's because processed foods often have a lot of sodium added to them. The average American consumes more than 3,400 milligrams of sodium per day, which is way above the recommended daily limit of 2,300 milligrams. Consuming too much sodium can also lead to weight gain, as well as high blood pressure and heart disease.

Finally, let's talk about artificial ingredients. Artificial sweeteners, preservatives, and flavours are often used to enhance the taste and extend the shelf life of processed foods. Unfortunately, these ingredients can disrupt the balance of hormones in your body and lead to weight gain. They can also negatively impact gut health, cause inflammation, and disrupt gut hormones, leading to weight gain.

It's crucial to be aware of the number of added sugars, sodium, and artificial ingredients in the food you buy. Reading food labels and making informed choices can help you avoid these harmful ingredients. The government also has a role to play in regulating the food industry and protecting consumers. By eating whole foods, cooking your own meals, and being mindful of what you're consuming, you can make healthier food choices and potentially avoid weight gain.

The Impact of Processed Foods On Health, Hormones, Metabolism and Gut Health

You may not realize it, but many processed foods are high in added sugars, sodium, and artificial ingredients that can cause some serious health problems.

Let's start with added sugars. You see, consuming too much added sugar can throw off your hormones, specifically insulin, which regulates your blood sugar levels. If you consume too much added sugar, your body can become less sensitive to insulin, leading to insulin resistance. This can increase your risk of developing type 2 diabetes and lead to weight gain, as your body struggles to burn fat.

Next, let's talk about sodium. Processed foods are often high in sodium, which can cause water retention, leading to weight gain and making it harder for your body to burn fat. High sodium levels can also affect the balance of hormones and put pressure on your kidneys, increasing your risk of high blood pressure and heart disease.

And finally, let's talk about artificial ingredients. These ingredients can cause inflammation, disrupt your gut hormones, and ultimately lead to weight gain. Your gut microbiome plays a critical role in regulating your metabolism and it's important to maintain a healthy gut to reduce inflammation and support overall health.

Unfortunately, processed foods often lack fiber, vitamins, and minerals that are important for healthy digestion and gut health. This can lead to digestive discomfort, constipation, and an overgrowth of harmful bacteria in the gut.

So, what can you do to protect your health? First, try to eat whole foods as much as possible and cook your own meals. Second, be sure to read food labels and look for added sugars, sodium, and artificial ingredients. This will help you make healthier food choices and avoid these harmful ingredients.

Choosing Whole Foods

Whole foods are foods that are minimally processed, close to their natural state, and are rich in nutrients like vitamins, minerals, and fiber. These foods include fruits, vegetables, whole grains, and lean proteins like chicken, fish, and eggs.

By incorporating whole foods into your diet, you'll be giving your body the essential nutrients it needs to function optimally. Fruits and vegetables, for example, are packed with antioxidants and phytochemicals that can help reduce inflammation and protect against chronic diseases.

Whole grains like quinoa and brown rice are great sources of fiber, which not only promotes feelings of fullness and improved digestion, but also helps regulate your metabolism. And don't forget about healthy fats! Foods like nuts, avocados, and olive oil provide healthy fats that are essential for maintaining optimal testosterone levels, improved absorption of vitamins A, D, and E, and a healthy weight.

On the other hand, processed foods are typically high in added sugars, sodium, artificial ingredients, and unhealthy fats, which can contribute to weight gain, hormone imbalances, and other health problems.

Here are examples of highly processed foods that are marketed as healthy but aren't:

- Granola bars
- Low-fat yogurt
- Energy bars
- Sushi [mainly the rice]
- 'high protein' options
- Processed meat substitutes
- Vegetable chips
- White bread, rice & pasta [stripped of nutrients]
- Sliced bread or 'low-calorie' bread
- Sweetened almond milk
- Fruit juice

- Packaged smoothie blends
- Multigrain breakfast cereals.
- Sports drinks
- Plant based milk alternatives
- Flavoured coffee drinks
- Frozen diet dinners
- Packaged gluten-free snacks
- Instant noodles
- Vegetable oils and spreads
- Dried fruit snacks
- Fat-free salad dressing
- Protein bars
- Processed cheese products.
- Ready-to-eat meals
- Flavoured water
- Packaged baked goods
- Low-carb snacks
- Instant soups
- Flavoured popcorn
- Sweetened breakfast cereals
- Pre-made dips and sauces.
- Processed snack bars

There are many more, but you get the idea! Just because they are low calorie doesn't mean they are good for you or will help you lose weight.

Whole foods, you'll be able to control your calorie intake more easily, as they are often lower in calories but more filling than processed foods. Plus, whole foods are abundant in fiber, which helps keep your digestion regular and supports a healthy gut.

When it comes to incorporating whole foods into your diet, it is important to start small and make gradual changes. Here are some tips that can help:

Plan ahead: Before you go food shopping, take some time to plan out your meals for the week. This will help you make better food choices and avoid last-minute decisions that may lead to unhealthy options.

Make a shopping list: Write down the foods you need for your meals and snacks so that you can focus on buying whole foods.

Try new fruits and vegetables: Experiment with different fruits [mostly low glycaemic choices] and vegetables that you haven't tried before. This can make eating healthy more interesting and enjoyable plus I recommend consuming 25-30 different colours a week to get the best spectrum of vitamins and minerals.

Cook at home: Cooking your own meals is a great way to control what you eat and ensure that you're eating whole foods.

Be mindful of portion sizes: It's easy to eat more than you need when you're eating processed foods, so be mindful of portion sizes when you're eating whole foods.

Keep healthy snacks on hand: Keep healthy snacks, such as fruits and vegetables, on hand so that you can grab something healthy when you're feeling hungry.

Incorporate healthy fats in your diet: Include healthy fats in your diet, such as avocado, nuts, seeds, and olive oil, as they are beneficial for hormones and weight loss.

Real food is the only ingredient: You should be able to see what you are eating and what is in it! Read the labels of the food products you buy, and make sure that the ingredients are whole foods and not processed. This will help you avoid consuming harmful additives and chemicals.

By choosing whole foods and incorporating them into your diet, you can improve your health and lose weight in a sustainable way.

Chapter 3: Re-thinking The Calorie Myth

Understanding Caloric Balance

So, you may have heard that weight loss is simply a matter of calories in and calories out, but, it's a little more complicated than that. While it's true that to lose weight you need to burn more calories than you consume, there are many other factors that can affect weight loss too.

One of the key things to keep in mind is the role of macronutrients, like protein, carbohydrates, and fats, in weight loss. Different types of food have different effects on your body, and they can impact your weight loss journey in different ways.

For instance, protein is a very filling macronutrient and can help you feel full for longer, making it easier to stick to a calorie-controlled diet. On the other hand, foods high in added sugars and processed carbs can trigger cravings and lead to overeating, making it harder for you to stick to your diet.

So, it's important to remember that not all calories are equal. A calorie from a donut is not the same as a calorie from broccoli.

The "calories in, calories out" model doesn't consider the important role that micronutrients, like vitamins and minerals, play in weight loss. These micronutrients are essential for overall health and can help regulate your metabolism, hormone production, and other bodily functions that impact your weight.

So, by eating a diet that is rich in micronutrients, you can give your body the support it needs to lose weight more easily.

Another factor that the "calories in, calories out" model neglects is the role of genetics and individual differences in weight loss. Some people may be more prone to storing fat or have a more efficient metabolism, making it harder for them to lose weight. It's also important to remember that all calories are not equal. The body reacts differently to different types of food, and this is known as the thermic effect of food. For example, protein has a higher thermic effect than carbohydrates or fat, meaning that your body must work harder to digest it, leading to greater calorie expenditure and weight loss.

When we try to restrict our calories, our body may respond in ways that make it harder to shed those extra pounds.

One of the ways our body responds is by slowing down our metabolism. This is a survival mechanism that our bodies have developed to conserve energy when food is scarce. So, even if we eat less, our body may still burn fewer calories, making weight loss more challenging.

Additionally, when we eat less, our body may store more fat. It does this to prepare for future periods of food scarcity, even if those periods never come. This can make it harder for us to lose weight, as our body is fighting against our efforts to reduce our calorie intake.

Lastly, it's important to think about your mindset when consuming low calorie foods.

You may think 'if I have a low fat snack, I can have more of it!' or you can 'squeeze' in a slice of chocolate cake, as you can see this just leads to more processed foods and weight gain.

So, as you can see, losing weight is not just about eating less. It's a complex process influenced by many factors, including our mindset, metabolism, hormones, and genetics. That's why it's important to focus on the quality of the food we eat, rather than just counting calories.

Set Point Weight & Self-Regulation

Have you ever heard of the 'set point weight theory'? It's the idea that your body has a preferred weight range that it feels most comfortable at, and it will naturally gravitate towards that weight. This weight can be influenced by things like your genetics, hormones, and metabolism.

The good news is that eating a high-quality diet can have a significant impact on your body's ability to regulate your weight and overall health. A diet that is filled with whole, nutrient-dense foods and is low in processed foods can help optimize your body's functions, promote weight loss, and even regulate your hormones.

An animal study by Nancy J. Rothwell an Michael J Stock (18) showed that animals that switched to a so called 'western diet' lost control of their intake, gained weight and became obese but when they switched to their 'regular correct food' their weight adjusted to previous levels.

It's clear that there is a strong correlation with eating high-quality food vs low-quality foods and how the body responds when they are consumed.

Hormones play a huge role in regulating your appetite, metabolism, and energy balance. By eating a diet that is high in protein and fiber, you can help regulate hormones like ghrelin and leptin, which are responsible for controlling your appetite. Additionally, eating an adequate amount of fiber can also help maintain a healthy gut microbiome, which has been linked to better weight management and overall health.

When you eat a high-quality diet, you are providing your body with the nutrients it needs to function properly. This can help boost your metabolism and improve your insulin sensitivity, which can promote weight loss and reduce the risk of diabetes. And because whole, nutrient-dense foods are more satisfying than processed foods, you'll feel full and satisfied, making it easier to stick to a calorie-restricted diet and achieve your weight loss goals.

Finally, by providing your body with the nutrients it needs, a high-quality diet can help improve the body's ability to self-regulate its weight. When your body is functioning optimally, it can better regulate its metabolism and energy balance, making it easier for you to lose weight and maintain a healthy weight in the long run.

Counting Calories & Trackers

One approach that you may have heard of is counting calories and using calorie trackers. However, counting calories and using calorie trackers can be a challenging task, even for professionals, and can be quite inaccurate for several reasons.

First, humans are not very good at estimating portion sizes and calorie counts. Studies have shown that people tend to significantly underestimate the number of calories they consume, which can make it difficult to accurately track calorie intake.

Another factor that makes it difficult to measure calorie intake is the inaccuracies in food labels. Food labels are required to list the number of calories per serving, but serving sizes listed on the label may not always reflect the amount of food that people typically consume. Additionally, food labels are not always accurate, and the calorie counts may be off by a significant amount.

Calorie trackers can also be inaccurate, as they may not always consider the specific characteristics of the food being consumed. For example, some calorie trackers may not consider the cooking method used or the specific brand of food being consumed.

Furthermore, calorie trackers are based on a system of averages that ignores the complexity of digestion, hunger, adherence, hormones, and other factors that can impact calorie intake and weight management.

Given these limitations, it's important to focus on habits and food quality, rather than counting calories. Instead of tracking calories, it's more important to focus on developing healthy eating habits such as eating a diet that is rich in whole, nutrient-dense foods, and limiting processed foods. Eating in a mindful way, paying attention to hunger and fullness cues, and focusing on nutrient density can help you achieve weight loss and maintain a healthy weight.

By focusing on developing healthy eating habits, you can avoid the inaccuracies and limitations of counting calories and using calorie trackers. This approach can help you achieve weight loss and maintain a healthy weight over time, and can be a much more effective and sustainable way to manage your weight compared to counting calories and using calorie trackers.

Do You Really Need Breakfast?

The idea that breakfast is the most important meal of the day has been challenged in recent years. Some experts believe that skipping breakfast and practising intermittent fasting can lead to benefits like weight loss and improved insulin sensitivity. This idea might sound tempting, especially if you have a sedentary job, but skipping breakfast may not be the best approach for everyone.

It's important to note that the conventional wisdom of breakfast being the most important meal was propagated largely by food companies. In today's world, most of us are already eating too much food, and skipping breakfast might just mean that we end up consuming a bigger dinner. Eating three meals a day is more than enough for most people.

Snacking and grazing throughout the day, as encouraged by many food companies, is not a healthy approach to weight loss. This kind of eating pattern can lead to overeating and a constant state of insulin release, which can result in weight gain and other health problems. Instead, focus on the quality and nutrient density of the food you eat, rather than the quantity.

Drinking plenty of water is also a key aspect of a healthy diet. Water can help control your appetite, increase feelings of fullness, and flush out toxins from your body. Staying hydrated is essential for your overall health and wellbeing.

Calorie counting and exercise alone may not be effective in achieving weight loss and maintaining a healthy weight, as per long-term studies. To be successful in losing weight and improving your overall health, it's important to take a holistic approach that considers other factors like stress, sleep and your lifestyle.

It's important to keep in mind that calorie counting and calorie trackers are based on a system of averages that ignores the complexity of digestion, hunger, adherence, hormones, and other biological and psychological factors. To truly achieve and maintain a healthy weight, it's important to adopt healthy habits and focus on the quality of the food you eat, rather than the quantity.

The Role of Nutrients

Nutrient density is a concept that helps us understand the relationship between the nutrients and calories in food. In simple terms, it refers to the amount of essential vitamins, minerals, and other nutrients in a food compared to the number of calories it provides. The goal is to find foods that provide a high amount of nutrients for every calorie consumed.

The importance of nutrient density in weight loss is well-established in the scientific community. When you consume a diet that is rich in nutrient-dense foods, you can lose weight, improve your overall health, and find the right balance for your body. This is because these foods are packed with essential nutrients and lower in calories, allowing you to eat fewer calories while still getting the nutrients your body needs.

Nutrient-dense foods are also known to be more satiating, meaning they keep you feeling full and satisfied for longer. This can help you reduce your appetite and cravings, making it easier to stick to a healthy diet.

One of the most crucial components of nutrient density is fiber. Fiber is a type of indigestible carbohydrate that helps to fill you up and keep you feeling satisfied. Foods high in fiber, such as fruits, vegetables, and whole grains, are more satiating than foods low in fiber, such as processed foods and sugary snacks. These foods also tend to be nutrient-dense, providing a variety of essential vitamins and minerals.

Another important aspect of nutrient density is the presence of micronutrients. Micronutrients are essential vitamins and minerals that our body needs in small amounts. This includes vitamins like vitamin C and vitamin A, and minerals like iron and calcium. These micronutrients play a critical role in maintaining our overall health and well-being.

The Impact of Satiety

You know how it is, when you're hungry, it's tough to resist snacking on junk food and overeating. That's why it's important to eat foods that will keep you full and satisfied for longer periods of time.

This is where protein comes in. Protein is a slow-digesting nutrient that will help you feel full for longer. Plus, it's important to keep your muscle mass in check when you're losing weight because muscle tissue burns more calories than fat tissue. Eating lean protein-rich foods such as fish, chicken, eggs, and legumes can help you with that.

Now, let's talk about processed foods. Unfortunately, these foods won't help you with weight loss and feeling full. They're often high in added sugars and unhealthy fats, which can cause a spike in blood sugar levels and increase hunger. Moreover, they're often low in fiber and protein, making it difficult to feel full and satisfied. The additives and preservatives in processed foods can also mess with your hunger and satiety hormone levels. On top of that, processed foods are usually high in calories and low in nutrients, which can lead to weight gain.

So, what should you focus on to promote satiety and support weight loss? Whole, nutrient-dense foods that are high in fiber and protein, like fruits and vegetables, whole grains, lean proteins, and healthy fats. This type of diet will not only help you feel full and satisfied but also support your weight loss journey.

The Importance of Timing

The way you eat, when you eat, and how often you eat all play a big role in regulating your energy balance and ultimately affecting your weight. That's why it's important to pay attention to meal timing and frequency.

First, let's talk about meal timing. Eating at consistent times throughout the day is a crucial aspect of weight loss. Research has shown that having a set eating schedule can improve your ability to regulate your energy balance and aid in weight loss. Consistent meal timing also helps regulate your body's circadian rhythm, which is important for overall health and metabolism. And not to mention, it can help you avoid overeating and snacking on unhealthy, high-calorie foods that can contribute to weight gain.

Now, let's talk about meal frequency. The traditional pattern is to eat three meals a day - breakfast, lunch, and dinner. But, there are other options like eating 4-6 smaller meals, or skipping a meal or two for weight loss. Eating more frequent, smaller meals throughout the day has been shown to regulate blood sugar levels and improve feelings of fullness. However, snacking and grazing all day can lead to weight gain, so it's important to find what approach works best for you.

You may have heard of Intermittent Fasting (IF). IF is a type of eating pattern where you alternate periods of eating with periods of fasting. Research has shown that it can be effective for weight loss by reducing overall calorie intake and improving insulin sensitivity. However, it's not for everyone, and it's always best to consult with a healthcare professional before starting any new eating pattern.

Another popular eating pattern for weight loss is Time-Restricted Eating (TRE). TRE involves eating only within a specific window of time each day, which can be as short as 4-6 hours or as long as 12-14 hours. The idea behind it is to reduce the number of hours per day during which you eat, reducing your overall calorie intake and improving your body's ability to burn fat. Studies have shown that TRE can lead to weight loss, improve insulin sensitivity, and cardiovascular health markers.

In conclusion, meal timing and frequency are important factors to consider in your weight loss journey. Eating at consistent times throughout the day, eating more frequent, smaller meals, and incorporating eating patterns such as Intermittent Fasting or Time-Restricted Eating can all aid in weight loss by helping regulate energy balance and improve feelings of fullness. However, it's important to keep in mind that what works for one person may not work for another, and it's always best to listen to your body and work with a healthcare professional if necessary.

Chapter 4: Transforming Your Mental Health

Understanding Emotional Eating

Let's talk about understanding emotional eating and how it affects your weight loss and mental health journey. Mental health and weight loss are closely intertwined, and it's essential to address both to be successful in losing weight.

Studies show that people who have a better understanding of their emotions and can manage stress are more likely to be successful in their weight loss efforts. Mental health issues like depression, anxiety, and stress can lead to weight gain and overeating, especially when food is used as a source of comfort. Some medications used to treat mental health conditions can also cause weight gain as a side effect. On the other hand, being overweight or obese can lead to poor mental health, as well as the physical limitations and health issues associated with it.

Here are some tips to help you overcome the effects of emotional eating and improve your mental health:

Identify your triggers: Journaling, therapy, or self-reflection can help you identify the underlying emotional triggers that lead to emotional eating.

Find alternative coping mechanisms: Once the triggers have been identified, find alternative coping mechanisms, such as exercise, therapy, or mindfulness practices, to address the underlying emotional distress. Practising yoga, meditation, or deep breathing can help reduce stress and anxiety and promote relaxation.

Practice mindful eating: Mindful eating means being present and fully engaged in the act of eating, paying attention to the taste, texture, and smell of the food, rather than eating mindlessly. Mindful eating can help you become more aware of your physical hunger and fullness cues, and make more intentional food choices.

Keep a food diary: Keeping a food diary can clarify patterns of emotional eating and help you make healthier food choices.

Seek professional help: If necessary, seek the help of a life coach, therapist, or counsellor to address underlying emotional issues and a nutritionist or dietitian to develop a healthy eating plan.

Exercise is also an important part of both mental health and weight loss. Regular physical activity has been shown to improve mood and reduce stress, as well as aid in weight loss. Mindfulness practices such as yoga and meditation can also be helpful in managing stress and improving mental health.

Overcoming Negative Self-Talk

Weight loss can be a tough journey, but with a positive mindset, healthy eating habits, and regular exercise, you can achieve your goals. However, negative self-talk can make it harder for you to reach your goals and even make your weight loss journey more challenging.

Negative self-talk refers to the negative thoughts and beliefs you have about yourself. These thoughts could be about your body, abilities, or personality. It could take the form of self-doubt, self-criticism, or self-blame. And unfortunately, it can impact your weight loss efforts in several ways, such as decreasing your motivation and self-esteem, increasing stress levels, and promoting negative thought patterns.

Identifying and Challenging Negative Thoughts

Awareness: Start by becoming aware of when negative self-talk occurs. Pay attention to your thoughts and emotions and recognize when negative thoughts arise.

Challenge: Once you have identified a negative thought, challenge it. Ask yourself if the thought is based on facts or if it's just a misinterpretation of reality.

Reframe: After challenging the thought, try to reframe it into a more positive statement. For example, instead of saying "I'll never be able to lose weight," reframe it to "I may struggle at times, but with effort and perseverance, I can reach my weight loss goals."

Practice gratitude: Practicing gratitude can help shift your focus from negative thoughts to the positive aspects of your life.

In conclusion, by being aware of your negative thoughts, challenging them, reframing them, practicing gratitude, and seeking support, you can overcome negative self-talk and achieve your weight loss goals. You got this!

Dealing With Negative States of Mind

I understand that life can get busy and responsibilities can pile up, making it difficult to focus on weight loss. But it's important to remember that taking care of yourself is just as important as taking care of your loved ones and responsibilities.

Dealing with negative states of mind such as procrastination, overwhelm, anxiety, and depression can make weight loss even harder. However, there are ways to overcome these challenges. To beat procrastination, it's important to set clear and specific goals, break tasks into manageable chunks, and create a schedule. It's also crucial to identify the root cause of procrastination and address it directly. Mindfulness and challenging negative thoughts can also help you overcome procrastination.

Anxiety and depression are a bit more complex, but there are still things you can do to improve your mood and reduce feelings of anxiety. Regular exercise, healthy eating, adequate sleep, and doing things you enjoy can all help. Mindfulness, learning relaxation techniques like deep breathing, and setting boundaries to reduce stress can also make a big difference.

Overwhelm can be caused by taking on too much, lack of control, or unrealistic expectations. To overcome it, prioritize tasks, delegate, or outsource where possible, and learn to say "no" to non-essential commitments. Taking regular breaks and practicing self-care are also important.

Remember, everyone's experience is unique, and what works for someone else may not work for you. Be kind and compassionate to yourself, and don't hesitate to seek professional help if needed. Surrounding yourself with a supportive network can help keep you motivated and accountable, and mindfulness can help you stay focused on your goals. And remember, setbacks are normal, so use them as opportunities to learn and grow.

n conclusion, weight loss is not just a physical ourney, it's a mental one as well.

Common Obstacles & Excuses

As a Dad, weight loss can seem like a daunting task with a lot of obstacles in the way. It's common to feel ike you don't have enough time, energy, or motivation o prioritize your health. However, with a few adjustments to your routine and mindset, you can overcome these challenges and achieve your weight loss goals.

Lack of Time: One of the biggest excuses for not having time for exercise or meal prep is a busy schedule. To combat this, try scheduling your workouts and meal planning in advance. Also, consider shorter, high-intensity workouts that you can fit into a busy day.

Lack of Energy: Feeling tired and run down can also make it difficult to focus on your weight loss journey. To increase your energy levels, make sure to get adequate sleep and adopt healthy habits like regular exercise and a nutritious diet. You can also reduce stress through mindfulness, yoga, or other stress-reduction techniques.

Lack of Motivation: Staying motivated can be a challenge, but setting specific, measurable, and achievable weight loss goals can help. Track your progress, celebrate your successes, and seek support from family, friends, or a coach to stay accountable and motivated.

Limited Access to Healthy Food: If you have limited access to healthy food options, try meal prepping in advance. You can also explore local farmer's market or food co-ops for fresh, healthy options.

Family Responsibilities: If you have young children, balancing family time with your weight loss journey can be a challenge. To overcome this, you can involve your children in your weight loss journey by exercising and eating healthy foods together. By setting a good example and leading by example, you can also inspire your family to adopt healthy habits.

In conclusion, by making time for exercise and healthy eating, managing stress, setting achievable goals, and seeking support, you can successfully lose weight and improve your overall health and well-being. Remember to be kind to yourself and celebrate your progress along the way.

Chapter 5: The Busy Dad's Guide to Exercise

I know you've got a lot on your plate, but trust me when I say that exercise should be at the top of your priority list. It's a critical aspect of maintaining good health, both physically and mentally.

Let's start with the physical benefits. Regular exercise can boost your heart health, lower your blood pressure, and reduce your risk of chronic illnesses like diabetes and heart disease. It also helps improve muscle and bone strength, keeping you injury-free and in shape.

Next, let's talk about stress management. Stress is a normal part of life, but when it becomes chronic, it can harm both your physical and mental health. Exercise can help combat stress by releasing endorphins, which will lift your mood and reduce anxiety. Plus, it can reduce cortisol levels, a stress hormone that can harm your health in many ways.

When it comes to mental health, exercise is a powerful tool to manage anxiety and depression. Regular physical activity can enhance your mood, lower anxiety, and depression, and even help prevent these conditions from developing. This is likely due to the release of endorphins and exercise's positive effects on the brain.

Exercise is also crucial for keeping your mind sharp. It's been proven to improve memory and concentration and can slow down age-related cognitive decline. Plus, regular exercise can boost your executive function, which is essential for handling complex tasks.

Lastly, exercise is important for overall well-being. It increases self-esteem, reduces feelings of loneliness and isolation, and enhances your quality of life.

So, there you have it, Dad. I hope this convinces you to make exercise a regular part of your routine. Your body and mind will thank you for it!

The Failure of Traditional Exercise Approaches

You know, for years, people have been told that if you just exercise enough, you'll lose weight and get in shape. But, the truth is that exercise is not as effective at burning calories as we think it is. In fact, it can even make weight loss harder by increasing hunger.

A common belief is that weight loss is just a matter of burning more calories than you consume. But, that's not the case. Our bodies are very adaptable and will adjust to increased physical activity by reducing energy spent on other tasks like inflammation and stress response. This is known as compensatory response.

A study of the Hadza people in Tanzania (19), who walk for miles every day foraging for food, shows this perfectly. Despite their high physical activity, they burned the same amount of energy as sedentary people in the West. This demonstrates that our bodies are designed to keep daily energy expenditure within a narrow window, regardless of how active we are.

Another study by Dr. Herman Pontzer (20), a professor of evolutionary anthropology at Duke University, suggests that exercise isn't the best tool for weight loss. He suggests that diet is the key and that the processed foods we eat today, with added oils and sugars, are designed to affect our brains in addictive ways. Therefore people who focus on exercise alone for weight loss often end up frustrated when they don't see results despite putting in a lot of effort.

Exercise does have many benefits, such as improving cardiovascular health, building muscle and bone density, and reducing the risk of chronic diseases. But, when it comes to weight loss, it's not as effective as we think. The best way to lose weight is to focus on diet and eat less because weight loss is primarily about calorie balance. The most effective way to reduce calorie intake is to control portion sizes and choose low-calorie foods.

Also, exercise can fuel hunger and make it harder to stick to a diet. When we exercise, our bodies release hormones such as ghrelin which increases appetite. This can lead to overeating and make it harder to stick to a calorie-controlled diet. Plus, muscle soreness from exercise can discourage people from continuing to exercise, making it harder to maintain an active lifestyle.

So, while exercise isn't the magic solution for weight loss, it's still an important part of a healthy lifestyle. To lose weight, focus on diet and eating less, rather than relying solely on exercise to burn calories. And, keep in mind that exercise can fuel hunger and make it harder to stick to a diet.

The Truth About Cardio

100% of the energy we receive comes from food, but up to 30% is the maximum we can burn through exercise, interesting right?

You probably already know that people often say cardio is important for weight loss because it burns a lot of calories. But, here's the truth - cardio is important for your overall health, but it's not as effective for weight loss as people think.

You would need to spend over 6 hours on the treadmill to burn 1 pound of fat if you didn't change your diet and you can easily 'eat back' the calories you burn after the session is complete, something that most people do!

Another thing to consider is that cardio can be boring, especially if you're doing it for a long time. That's why a lot of people give up on their weight loss goals because they can't stick to a cardio routine. And it's also worth mentioning that cardio can be tough to sustain in the long run, as it can lead to burnout and injuries from overuse.

But here's some good news - you don't have to rely solely on cardio to lose weight. Combining cardio with resistance training is a great way to lose weight, improve your overall health, and build muscle. And, when you have more muscle, your body burns more calories even when you're not working out.

In conclusion, cardio is a crucial part of overall health and fitness, but it has its limitations when it comes to weight loss. To reach your weight loss goals, you'll get the best results by combining cardio with other forms of exercise, such as resistance training.

The Benefits of Resistance and Circuit Training

If you're looking for long-term weight loss results, then resistance and circuit training are the way to go. These forms of exercise focus on building and maintaining muscle mass, which is key to a sustainable weight loss journey.

Here's why: unlike cardio, which only burns calories, resistance, and circuit training increase muscle mass and thus your metabolism. This means your body burns more calories, even when you're not working out. And the more muscle you have, the more calories your body burns, even at rest.

Just 1 lb of muscle burns 50 calories a day without exercise! So you can increase your metabolic rate without having to run yourself into the ground.

Not only that, resistance and circuit training also increase testosterone levels in your body, which is a hormone that helps with weight loss. It increases muscle mass and decreases body fat, making it a key player in your weight loss journey.

But don't worry, you don't have to turn into a bodybuilder to see results. Maintaining muscle mass while shedding body fat is the goal, and this can be achieved through circuit training at home or at the gym, with or without weights. I know how tough it can be to get to the gym with a busy schedule, so many of my clients and I train from the comfort of our own homes for about 30 minutes, 3 days a week, and we've seen great results.

It's important to remember that trying to build muscle and lose weight at the same time is not sustainable or will not produce the best results. Focus on losing weight first, and then incorporating resistance and circuit training to maintain muscle mass. This approach will lead to sustainable weight loss and improved overall health and fitness.

In conclusion, while cardio is a good start, resistance and circuit training offer a more effective and sustainable approach to weight loss. Build and maintain muscle mass, increase your metabolism, and improve your overall health and fitness. And don't forget, weight loss is also about your diet, so make sure to fuel your body with the right nutrients.

Build your metabolism and body with exercise, and lose weight with your diet.

How To Make It Sustainable (and Save Time)

When it comes to losing weight and improving overall health, exercise plays a crucial role. However, many people struggle with making exercise a sustainable part of their lives. Whether it's due to lack of time, lack of motivation, or burnout, it can be difficult to stick with an exercise routine for the long term.

It's a complete myth that you must exercise for hours every day, this belief will hold you back due to 'all or nothing thinking'.

Will 1 salad a day not make a difference?

Will a 20 min jog not make a difference?

Will 1 set of squats not make a difference?

Of course it will, any time you take action you produce a result, but sitting on the fence waiting for the perfect time to be 'all-in' and thinking 'what's the point' is a limiting belief you need to forget about.

One key to making exercise sustainable is to focus on time-efficiency. Instead of trying to squeeze in hours of exercise each day, aim for shorter, more intense workouts that can be done in a shorter period. For example, a 30-minute circuit training session or a brisk 20-minute walk can be just as effective as a longer workout, but without the time commitment.

Another important aspect of making exercise sustainable is consistency. It's better to do a short workout 3 times a week for a year, than to try to exercise every day for a few weeks and then give up.

Building exercise into your daily routine can also make it more sustainable. For example, taking a lunchtime walk, getting off the train or bus a stop early, or parking your car a bit further from work can all add up to a significant amount of activity over time.

Additionally, it's important to focus on building and maintaining muscle, rather than trying to burn calories. Building muscle can help boost metabolism, which can lead to sustainable weight loss over time. And forget working your abs, working out full body burns more calories than isolated exercises, which is what will give you a flatter belly. That's why a squat, which is a big compound lift, is better than a bicep curl when it comes to getting lean and mean. My preference is always to work full body for this reason.

However, it's important to note that when trying to lose weight, it's not sustainable or effective to try to build muscle at the same time. Instead, focus on maintaining muscle mass while reducing caloric intake to lose weight.

Finally, to make exercise sustainable it's also important to make it enjoyable. Finding activities that you enjoy, such as swimming, hiking, or playing a sport, can make it more likely that you'll stick with it in the long term.

In conclusion, making exercise sustainable requires a combination of time efficiency, consistency, focus on muscle building and maintenance, and making it enjoyable.

By incorporating these elements into your exercise routine, you can achieve sustainable weight loss and improve your overall health.

Chapter 6: Goals, Momentum & Motion

Discover The Real Goal

When it comes to losing weight, you must be real with yourself. This is not always a simple task in todays world where people have become more disconnected from their true feelings and emotions because they don't take the time to check in with themselves and practise enough 'self-care'.

To add to this, being constantly 'in your head' with many responsibilities and the distraction of technologies such as Netflix, social media and the media in general doesn't help.

So take a moment to check in with yourself and do it regularly!

A lot of people start a weight loss journey with the goal of simply losing weight or getting fit, but that won't cut it in the long run. You need to dig deep and find the reason why you really want to get fit.

Think about what getting fit will bring you. Will it give you more energy to keep up with the kids? Will it improve your confidence and self-esteem? Will it lower your risk of chronic diseases and improve your overall health? Whatever your reason may be, make sure you have a clear, specific goal that you keep in mind.

When things get tough, it's easy to give up. That's why it's important to have an emotional connection to your goal. It'll help you push through the tough days and stay motivated.

Imagine if you don't change things. How will your health, career, family, and future be affected? This should be a powerful motivator for you to make the necessary changes in your life to achieve your weight loss goals.

Forget the fad diets and quick fixes. Sustainable weight loss comes from finding a lifestyle that you can stick to long-term. This means making small, maintainable changes like incorporating more whole foods into your diet, finding ways to move your body throughout the day, and setting realistic goals.

And remember, weight loss isn't just about the number on the scale. Building muscle and getting stronger is just as important, and it'll help increase your metabolism and make it easier to maintain your weight loss in the long run.

In conclusion, successful weight loss comes from finding your inner purpose, setting realistic goals, and making sustainable lifestyle changes. It won't be easy, but with the right mindset and emotional drive, you can achieve your goals and improve your overall health and well-being.

Goals, Momentum & Motion

Setting Goals

Are you ready to make some positive changes in your life and become the best version of yourself? Great! Let's start by setting some goals.

First, think about what your long-term vision is for yourself. It could be something like feeling more energetic, being able to play with your kids without feeling winded, or even fitting into those old clothes that have been sitting in your closet. Whatever it is, make sure it's something that motivates and inspires you.

Next, let's break down that big goal into smaller, more manageable pieces. For example, if your long-term vision is to fit into your old clothes, a good first step might be to set a goal to lose 10 pounds in the next month. This makes your goal more specific, measurable, and achievable.

Remember, it's important to make sure your goals are **SMART:** specific, measurable, attainable, relevant, and time-bound. Try to avoid unrealistic expectations and focus on progress, not perfection!

Also, it's important to also monitor other aspects of progress as part of a healthy lifestyle, this can be how your clothes fit, how you feel, comments from family, friends, and colleagues and even your consistency and effort in your journey.

This will keep you focused and motivated as you work towards achieving your goals.

Creating Momentum

When it comes to creating momentum, it's important to start slow and steady. You don't want to jump into something too quickly and get discouraged, especially if you're a busy Dad with a lot of responsibilities. Starting small and gradually increasing the difficulty level will not only help you avoid feeling overwhelmed, but it'll also help you get a better understanding of what works best for you.

As you progress, it's crucial to focus on one goal at a time. The human mind can only process so much information at once, and if you try to tackle multiple things at once, you're likely to become easily distracted and lose sight of your main goal. By focusing on one thing at a time, you can give it your full attention and make real progress.

Another important aspect of creating momentum is to celebrate the small wins along the way. We often get so caught up in the big picture that we forget to acknowledge the progress we've made. Celebrating the small wins, no matter how small, will give you a sense of accomplishment and keep you motivated. It's a great way to reinforce positive behaviour and remind yourself of the progress you've made so far. And as you continue to make progress, it'll build momentum that will carry you towards your bigger goals.

Remember, creating momentum is a process and it takes time. But if you stay focused, stay motivated and celebrate the small wins, you'll be well on your way to achieving your goals. And if you ever need a push, just remember why you started and keep pushing forward. You got this!

Motion

Let's dive into how to get in motion and make it stick.

First, let's create a schedule that works for you. I understand as a busy Dad, it can be challenging to find time for yourself. But setting aside a specific time each day for exercise and healthy eating can make it easier to stick to. Try to schedule it at the same time each day to form a habit.

Next, let's make it convenient and easy to stick to your plan. This means finding ways to make healthy choices accessible and simple. For example, you can keep healthy snacks in your car, pack your gym bag the night before, or lay out your workout gear so you're ready to go in the morning. The goal is to remove any obstacles that might prevent you from sticking to your plan.

Another great way to stay motivated is by finding an accountability partner. This can be a friend, family member, or even an online community within a paid coaching programme. Having someone to check in with, hold you accountable, and cheer you on can be a great motivator, also working with a coach can give you the expertise and informed guidance to overcome roadblocks as they present themselves and help you get results faster than you would alone.

Significant changes take time, and there will be ups and downs along the way. But with a well-defined goal, a plan, and a support system, you can achieve your goals. Remember, everyone's journey is different, and it's important to find a plan that works for you and your lifestyle. With dedication and a positive attitude, you'll be on your way to a happier, healthier life.

Patience, Consistency & Adapting

It's completely normal to feel overwhelmed by the thought of making changes to your health and fitness, but being outside of your comfort zone is where the magic happens! But don't worry, it's totally achievable with some patience, consistency, and a willingness to adapt.

Truth is we live in a world of instant gratification and quick-fix mindsets, but lasting change is never as simple as that and you wouldn't truly appreciate your positive changes if you didn't have to work for them! First, let's talk about patience. I know, we all want instant results, but true success is a journey, not a destination. It's important to remember that progress takes time, and setbacks are just opportunities to learn and grow. So, instead of getting discouraged when progress is slow, focus on the progress you have made so far and celebrate your small wins. That will help you stay motivated and patient.

Next, consistency is key. You need to make healthy habits a regular part of your daily routine by committing to a regular exercise routine, sticking to a healthy diet, and making time for self-care. A good way to do this is by creating a schedule or routine and sticking to it. That way, you'll be able to develop the habits you need to maintain a healthy lifestyle.

Finally, adaptability is also important. Your approach may need to change as you progress, so be open to new ideas, new forms of support and change when necessary. Don't be afraid to ask for help or seek out new forms of support. Results should be seen as feedback, not good or bad, but as an opportunity to learn and grow.

So, don't be discouraged by the thought of making changes. With patience, consistency, and the willingness to adapt, you can create a healthy and fulfilling lifestyle that works for you and your family. Celebrate your successes, no matter how small they may be, and remember to focus on the journey, not the destination. With these principles in mind, you'll be able to achieve your goals and become the best version of yourself.

Chapter 7: Sustaining Your Weight Loss: A Lifetime Approach

I want to talk to you about how to make sustainable weight loss a part of your lifestyle.

Weight loss can feel like a never-ending journey, but it doesn't have to be that way. The key to success is making changes that you can stick with for the long haul. Sure, crash diets and extreme exercise routines might help you shed some pounds quickly, but they're not realistic or healthy in the long run. What you need to focus on is making healthy changes that you can easily integrate into your daily routine and maintain for the rest of your life.

One of the most crucial things to keep in mind is to not stress about being perfect. It's easy to get caught up in trying to do everything right, but the truth is, nobody is perfect. Instead of striving for perfection, aim to make progress and learn from your mistakes. Every small step you take towards a healthier lifestyle is a step in the right direction.

Making changes gradually is another essential part of sustainable weight loss. Trying to change everything at once can be overwhelming and hard to stick with. Start by making small changes to your routine, like adding a daily walk or swapping processed snacks for fruit. Over time, these small changes will add up and you'll be able to see significant results.

One of the best ways to make weight loss a lifetime habit is to focus on developing healthy habits. Habits are formed through repetition, and by establishing healthy habits, you'll be able to maintain a healthy lifestyle for the rest of your life. This means committing to a regular exercise routine, eating a balanced diet, and taking time for self-care. Whether it's a daily walk, a healthy meal, or a relaxing bubble bath, make sure you're taking care of yourself.

Remember, weight loss is a journey, not a destination. Take it one step at a time and focus on making changes that you can stick with for the long haul.

Understanding Plateaus and Why They Happen

let's talk about a common challenge that many people face on their weight loss journey: plateaus. I know, it can be discouraging when you're putting in the effort but not seeing progress on the scale. But, it's important to understand that weight loss plateaus are a normal part of the process and can happen for a variety of reasons.

One reason is a hormonal imbalance. Hormones play a crucial role in regulating your metabolism, appetite, and body weight. When they are out of balance, it can impact your weight loss journey. Hormonal imbalances can be caused by stress, poor sleep, or even medical conditions.

Another reason is a lack of variety in your diet and exercise routine. When you do the same thing repeatedly, your body becomes used to it and it becomes less effective. To keep making progress, it's important to switch things up and try new exercises and foods. Experimenting with new recipes, incorporating strength training into your workout routine, or trying a new form of exercise can all help prevent weight loss plateaus.

Emotional eating is also a common reason for weight loss plateaus. When you eat in response to emotions like stress, boredom, or sadness, it's easy to overeat and make unhealthy food choices. To overcome emotional eating, it's important to address the underlying emotional issues that are driving it. This may mean working with a therapist to identify and manage stressors in your life, practicing mindfulness, or finding alternative coping mechanisms for difficult emotions.

Mental plateaus can also be a roadblock in your weight loss journey. When you hit a mental roadblock, it can feel like you're not making progress and it can be easy to lose motivation. To overcome this, it's important to reframe your thinking and focus on progress, not perfection. Remind yourself of your goals, celebrate your victories, no matter how small, and seek support from family and friends.

In conclusion, weight loss plateaus are normal and can be caused by a variety of factors, including hormonal imbalances, lack of variety in diet and exercise, and emotional eating. To overcome plateaus, it's important to understand the underlying cause and take steps to address it. Whether that means trying new exercises, experimenting with new foods, or seeking support from a qualified Coach, know that you're not alone and that with determination and persistence, you can continue on your weight loss journey.

Staying Motivated

I know you're always on the go and trying to balance work, family and taking care of yourself. But, don't worry, I have some tips for you to stay motivated on your weight loss journey.

First, finding an accountability partner can really help. This could be a friend, family member, or even an online support group. Sharing your progress and struggles with someone can provide the support and encouragement you need to keep going.

It's also important to make time for yourself. You don't have to sacrifice your health just because you're busy. Find a few minutes each day to focus on your weight loss goals, like taking a walk during your lunch break or doing a quick workout at home before the kids wake up.

Incorporating physical activity into your daily routine can also be a big motivator. Try taking the stairs instead of the elevator, or make it more structured by going to the gym or joining a sports league.

Healthy eating can be a challenge when you're short on time, but there are ways to make it more convenient. Meal prepping on the weekends, having healthy snacks on hand, or ordering healthy meals from a meal delivery service can all help.

And, don't forget to reward yourself for your progress. Achieving weight loss goals is hard work, so buy yourself a treat or treat yourself to a massage.

It's okay if things don't always go as planned, just be flexible and adapt. If a workout or meal plan doesn't work out, don't beat yourself up, just try again tomorrow.

Remember why you started this journey in the first place, whether it's to be a healthier role model for your kids, improve your health, or feel better in your own skin. Keeping this end goal in mind can help you stay motivated.

A coaching program can also provide a lot of support and guidance. Your coach can help you set goals, create a plan, and provide the tools and resources you need to succeed. Successful people have mentors to guide them and I see many Dads initially tell themselves 'I can do it all myself' whilst struggling to create lasting change, but that's just ego and pride getting in the way, assuming you have the same level of experience, knowledge and tools as a qualified coach who has made this their profession is a mistake, invest in yourself and achieve your goals faster.

Joining an online community of people who are also on a weight loss journey can provide support and encouragement. Share your progress, ask questions, and offer advice to others, paid is always better than free not because of the quality of the people but the quality of the structure and leadership available, plus you always place a higher value on what you pay for vs what is free, so this is an extra reason to succeed and implement,

And finally, consistency is key. By sticking to your plan and making healthy choices most of the time, you'll be more likely to see results and stay motivated.

So, there you have it, 10 tips for staying motivated on your weight loss journey. Just remember, it's not going to be easy, but with these tips and some determination, you'll be able to reach your goals.

Taking Full Ownership

As a busy overweight dad, life can be a real challenge sometimes. With all the responsibilities and demands from work, family, and personal life, it's easy to feel like you're just going through the motions, with little control over the outcome. But the truth is, you have much more power over your life than you might realize. The key to unlocking this power is to take full ownership of your results.

Taking ownership means that you understand that you are responsible for creating the life you want, not just a victim of circumstance. You're the one in charge, and you can make changes to your life when things aren't working out. This shift in perspective can be life-changing, as it gives you the power to create new opportunities for yourself and your family.

One of the first steps in taking ownership is to adopt a growth mindset. This is the belief that you can improve and change through effort and learning. It's the opposite of a fixed mindset, which is the belief that you are stuck with the abilities and characteristics you have. With a growth mindset, you're open to new possibilities, and you're willing to put in the work to achieve your goals. This mindset is crucial, as it will help you to overcome obstacles and challenges that may come your way.

Another important aspect of taking ownership is understanding that change takes time and effort. It's not going to happen overnight, and it's important to be patient with yourself. Celebrate small wins along the way, as every step you take towards your goal is one step closer to achieving it. Remember, progress is progress, no matter how small.

The journey of achieving your goals is just as important as the destination. It's about becoming the best version of yourself, not just reaching a certain number on the scale, or hitting a certain income level. By focusing on the person you want to become, you'll be more likely to achieve your goals and create a life that's truly fulfilling for you and your family.

In conclusion, taking ownership of your results and life is essential for you as a busy overweight dad. It means understanding that you have the power to change things when they're not working for you, adopting a growth mindset, focusing on becoming the person you want to be, being patient, celebrating small wins, setting realistic goals, and surrounding yourself with supportive people. Change takes time and effort, but with determination and hard work, you can achieve anything you set your mind to. So, take control of your life, and make the changes you want to see. You have the power to create the life you want, and you can do it!

Chapter 8: Conclusion and Thoughts

As a fellow busy dad, it has been an honour to share with you my knowledge and experience through this book. The journey towards achieving your weight loss goals is not an easy one, but I hope that the information and strategies provided in this book have been valuable to you.

Thank you for taking the time to invest in yourself and your health. You are taking the first step towards a healthier, happier life, and that is something to be celebrated.

Throughout this book, we have explored the various factors that contribute to weight gain, including biological, psychological, and environmental factors, as well as the impact of diet trends and the changes brought about by the COVID-19 pandemic. We have also delved into the truth about processed foods, the role of calories in weight gain, and provided strategies for improving your mental health and overcoming emotional eating and negative self-talk.

We have also discussed the importance of making exercise sustainable and effective, and provided tips for setting and achieving weight loss goals that will last a lifetime.

I'd like to acknowledge and thank all my clients who have worked with me over the years. Their dedication and commitment has made me successful as a coach, and I am grateful for the opportunity to help them transform their health, body, and lives.

Now, it's time for you to act and make lasting changes. Use the tools and knowledge you have gained from this book to create the life you want. If you have any questions or would like to discuss your goals in more detail, don't hesitate to reach out.

Remember, you have the power to take ownership of your results and create a life that is truly fulfilling for you and your family. You can do it, Dad!

And for more information, visit the link below to our website, which has links to other valuable resources such as the podcast, our blog, YouTube, social media channels, and our coaching program.

In service,

Coach Stefano Chiriaco

Email: Stefano@ultimatedadtransformation.com
Website: www.UltimateDadTransformation.com

REFERENCES USED

(1) https://www.theguardian.com/society/2022/may/19/more-than-42m-uk-adults-will-be-overweight-by-2040

(2) https://www.bhf.org.uk/what-we-do/news-from-the-bhf/contact-the-press-office/facts-and-figures

(3) https://www.mind.org.uk/information-support/types-of-mental-health-problems/mental-health-problems-introduction/about-mental-health-problems/

(4) https://nhsfunding.info/mental-health/a-39-increase-in-child-referrals-for-mental-health-care-in-england-in-a-year/

(5) https://www.mayoclinic.org/diseases-conditions/diabetes/in-depth/insulin-and-weight-gain/art-20047836

(6) https://www.health.harvard.edu/staying-healthy/why-people-become-overweight

(7) https://www.health.harvard.edu/staying-healthy/do-gut-bacteria-inhibit-weight-loss

(8) https://www.health.harvard.edu/staying-healthy/why-stress-causes-people-to-overeat

(9) https://www.ncbi.nlm.nih.gov/pmc/articles/PMC5644966/

(10) https://www.ncbi.nlm.nih.gov/pmc/articles/PMC8717738/

(11) https://www.ncbi.nlm.nih.gov/pmc/articles/PMC1373635/

(12) https://pubmed.ncbi.nlm.nih.gov/33341313/

(13) https://www.ncbi.nlm.nih.gov/pmc/articles/PMC7434327/

(14) https://www.ncbi.nlm.nih.gov/pmc/articles/PMC8204767/

(15) https://www.thelancet.com/article/S0140-6736(19)30041-8/fulltext

(16) https://www.grandviewresearch.com/industry-analysis/dietary-supplements-market

(17) https://www.newfoodmagazine.com/news/142469/junk-food-europe/

(18) https://www.nature.com/articles/281031a0

(19) https://www.scientificamerican.com/article/the-exercise-paradox/

(20) https://gsas.harvard.edu/news/stories/colloquy-podcast-why-exercising-more-may-not-help-you-lose-weight

Printed in Great Britain
by Amazon

20242568R00061